# Managing Conduct Disorder in Children

*Evidence-Based Practical Strategies and Interventions for Creating Supportive Learning Environments, Positive Behavioural Change and Effective Treatment*

I0082508

## Michele L. Valdez

Introducing the exclusive and captivating world of Michele L. Valdez. Immerse yourself in the timeless elegance and creativity that defines our brand. Experience the unparalleled craftsmanship and attention to detail that sets us apart. Discover the essence of sophistication and style with our exquisite collection.

Copyright © 2024 Michele L. Valdez

Experience the exclusivity of our copyrighted content. Introducing an extraordinary publication that captivates the mind and sparks inspiration. This masterpiece is protected by the highest standards of copyright law. Reproduction, distribution, or transmission in any form or by any means is strictly prohibited without the prior written permission of the esteemed publisher. However, in the realm of critical reviews and select non-commercial uses, brief quotations may be embraced. Unlock the power of knowledge while respecting the rights of the visionary creators.

# Table of Contents

# Preface

Step into a world where challenges are transformed into conquerable feats and obstacles become mere stepping stones. Behold, a radiant beacon of hope that illuminates the path for parents, educators, and mental health professionals alike. Step into a world where the power of comprehension merges seamlessly with decisive steps, where wisdom blossoms into personal empowerment, and where each turn of the page unveils a fresh chapter in the epic journey of healing and self-development. Get ready to embark on an extraordinary and life-changing journey that is truly one-of-a-kind. Let our groundbreaking books, meticulously created with unwavering passion, precision, and a clear sense of purpose, be your guide.

Imagine this: a devoted parent standing at the crossroads, bravely navigating the intricate challenges of raising a child with conduct disorder. Experience the overwhelming weight of uncertainty as it bears down heavily upon you. Embark on a thrilling quest for answers that feels like navigating a treacherous labyrinth without the guidance of a map. Introducing "Managing Conduct Disorder in Children" - your guiding light in overcoming fear and finding solutions.

Embark on a remarkable journey as you delve into the captivating pages of this extraordinary book. Within its covers, you will unearth a wealth of invaluable insights, ingenious strategies, and indispensable practical tools meticulously crafted to empower you on your noble path of parenthood. Discover the secrets of understanding conduct disorder like never before. Unlock the power to create customized action plans that perfectly suit your child's individual needs. With this book by your side, you'll have an unwavering ally to guide you through the ups and downs of parenting, helping you conquer every challenge and celebrate every triumph.

Are you an educator or mental health professional? If so, you have been entrusted with the incredibly important responsibility of molding young minds and fostering their limitless potential. Introducing a group of students struggling with conduct disorder, the journey ahead may appear veiled in uncertainty. Discover the captivating world of "Conduct Disorder Decoded: Unraveling the Puzzle for Educators and Clinicians." Immerse yourself in this enlightening masterpiece that will leave you spellbound. Prepare to unlock the secrets and gain invaluable insights into the intricate realm of conduct disorder. Don't miss out on this must-read for educators and clinicians alike. Enter now and embark on a journey of knowledge and understanding.

Introducing our revolutionary guide that will empower you with the essential knowledge, cutting-edge tools, and game-changing strategies to effortlessly cultivate inclusive and supportive learning environments. With our expert guidance, you will unlock the potential for every student to not just succeed, but to truly thrive. Discover the secrets to understanding the intricate dynamics of conduct disorder and unlock the power to implement evidence-based interventions in your very own classroom. With this book in your hands, you hold the key to making a profound and lasting difference in the lives of your students.

Discover the unparalleled qualities that make this book truly stand out from the competition. Discover the extraordinary wealth of knowledge nestled within the pages of this remarkable book. Prepare to be captivated by the unparalleled clarity of its insights. But it doesn't stop there. Brace yourself for the transformative power that this book possesses, as it has the remarkable ability to ignite change and inspire tremendous growth. Get ready to embark on a journey like no other. Prepare to be captivated as you immerse yourself in a captivating narrative that will take you on a transformative voyage of self-discovery, unwavering resilience, and unparalleled empowerment. With every page you turn, you'll transcend the mere boundaries of written language, delving into a world where the power of words knows no limits.

Get ready to embark on a transformative journey driven by boundless compassion, groundbreaking innovation, and an unshakeable faith in the limitless potential of each and every person. Join the movement today! Unlock the power of transformation by taking that crucial first step towards a brighter future. Embrace the unparalleled wisdom that lies within the pages of this groundbreaking guide, and embark on a journey of self-discovery and personal growth. Are you a parent in need of solace and guidance? Or perhaps a professional with a burning desire to make a difference? Look no further! This incredible book is here to provide you with a roadmap to transformation and serve as a beacon of hope in a world filled with challenges. Get ready to embark on a life-changing journey!

Step into the magnificent tapestry of life, where each journey unfolds with unparalleled uniqueness, and every path is adorned with captivating twists and turns. Amidst the swirling chaos and ever-shifting uncertainty, there is a steadfast force that remains unwavering: the indomitable power that resides within each and every one of us. It is this power that enables us to transcend adversity and wholeheartedly embrace the boundless potential that lies within. Embark on an extraordinary journey with this book as your trusted guide. Discover the profound truth that the power to transform resides not in the destination, but in the very essence of the journey itself. Embrace the boundless opportunities that await you, seize the present moment, and embark on a transformative journey of self-empowerment, profound enlightenment, and ceaseless exploration.

As we reach the end of this incredible journey, let us take a moment to contemplate the immense influence of our combined endeavors. Within the captivating pages of this extraordinary book, we have embarked on an awe-inspiring journey of empowerment, enlightenment, and transformation. It is a journey that is ignited by an unwavering belief in the limitless potential that resides within each and every individual.

Dare to dream, dear reader, and unlock the limitless possibilities that await you. Imagine a world where knowledge conquers ignorance, where empathy rises above challenges, and where every person has the chance to flourish. Join us on an extraordinary voyage of self-empowerment, profound enlightenment, and boundless potential. Discover the true essence of life, where it's not the final destination that shapes our identity, but the extraordinary voyage we embark upon to reach it.

# Introduction

Unleash your potential with the ultimate handbook for comprehending and skilfully handling conduct disorder in children. Introducing "Managing Conduct Disorder in Children" - an extraordinary resource crafted by the esteemed child psychologist, Michele L. Valdez. Prepare to embark on a transformative journey as Valdez seamlessly blends her expert knowledge, invaluable strategies, and genuine empathy to empower parents, caregivers, and educators in confidently navigating the intricate world of conduct disorder. Brace yourself for a groundbreaking experience that will leave you equipped with the tools and wisdom needed to tackle this challenge with unwavering confidence and unwavering compassion.

## _Discover the Power of Unlocking the Key to Positive Change_

Experience the transformative power of Dr. [Author's Name]'s unparalleled empathy and expertise as they unravel the complexities of conduct disorder. Discover a comprehensive roadmap that will guide you towards nurturing your child's healthy development and forging deep, meaningful connections. Say goodbye to confusion and hello to a brighter future. Discover the ultimate guide that empowers you with the essential tools and knowledge to identify early warning signs, implement evidence-based interventions, and foster positive behavior while enhancing family dynamics. This comprehensive resource is your key to nurturing a harmonious and thriving family environment.

## *Introducing Practical Solutions for Real-World Challenges*

Uncover groundbreaking strategies for effectively handling defiance, aggression, and impulsivity, specifically designed to cater to your child's individual needs and exceptional strengths. Discover the power of insightful case studies, engaging interactive exercises, and time-tested parenting strategies. Unlock the secrets to effective communication, boundary setting, and conflict resolution. Empower yourself to create a supportive and nurturing environment where your child can truly thrive.

## *Unlocking the Potential of Parents, Revolutionizing Lives*

Introducing "Managing Conduct Disorder in Children"—a powerful resource that goes beyond a mere guidebook. Packed with empathy, wisdom, and practical advice, this invaluable tool serves as a lifeline for families bravely navigating the challenging waters of conduct disorder. Introducing an empowering resource that will be your guiding light through any challenges you may face - whether it's at home, in school, or within your community. This invaluable resource offers hope and guidance, ensuring that you never feel alone on your journey.

## _Embark on a journey towards a radiant future for your precious child._

Discover the key to unlocking a world of positive change today with the groundbreaking guide, "Managing Conduct Disorder in Children."

# Chapter 1

## Conduct Disorder: What Is It?

Conduct Disorder is a behavioral condition often identified in young individuals. It is characterized by antisocial behavior that disregards the rights of others and societal norms for their age group. From irresponsibility to delinquent behaviors like truancy or walking away, breaking the rights of others through fraud, and showing physical hostility towards pets or others like assault or rape. These behaviors can occur together at times, but they can also happen separately.

### What Leads to Conduct Disorder?

Various factors are believed to play a role in the development of Conduct Disorder, making it a complex issue with multiple contributing causes.

Neuropsychological testing reveals that children with Conduct Disorders may experience difficulties in the frontal lobe of their brain, affecting their ability to plan, avoid harm, and learn from negative experiences. Genetic factors play a role in childhood character development, leading to potential behavioral issues in children perceived as eccentric. Children growing up in challenging home environments are more likely to develop Conduct Disorders, although it can be found across all socioeconomic groups. Delinquency can be influenced by cultural issues and rejection from peer groups. Being in a lower socioeconomic position remains linked to Conduct Disorders. Children who display delinquent and intense behaviors have unique cognitive and mental profiles when compared to children with other mental health conditions and control groups. These factors impact children's interactions with others.

## Who suffers from Conduct Disorder?

Boys are more commonly affected by the disorder than girls. Children diagnosed with Conduct Disorders often experience additional psychiatric issues that can contribute to the development of Conduct Disorder. Conduct Disorders are on the rise in contemporary society, affecting people of all races, cultures, and economic backgrounds.

# Signs of Conduct Disorder

Many symptoms observed in children with Conduct Disorder can also appear in children who do not have this disorder. Yet, in kids diagnosed with Conduct Disorder, these behaviors occur often and impact their education, school performance, and social relationships.

Here are the common symptoms of Conduct Disorder. Nevertheless, each child may encounter these symptoms in a unique way. Here are the four symptoms:

- Assertiveness

- Being aggressive can lead to physical issues for both the individual and those in their vicinity.

- Intimidating conduct.

- Bullying.

- Physical altercations.

- Being cruel to others or animals.

- Utilization of weapon(s).

- Engaging in non-consensual sexual activities such as rape or molestation.

**Behavior that causes harm**

Examples of Destructive Conduct may involve Vandalism and intentional harm to property.

## *Deception*

Deception can manifest in various ways:

- Deception.

- Stealing.

- Stealing from a store.

- Debt default.

## *Breaking the rules*

Breaking the usual rules of behavior or age-appropriate standards could include:

1. Truancy (leaving college prematurely).

2. Moving on.

3. Pranks.

4. Causing trouble.

5. Engaging in sexual activity at a young age.

Conduct Disorder symptoms may resemble those of other medical conditions or behavioral issues. It's important to consult your child's doctor for a proper medical diagnosis.

## How is Conduct Disorder Diagnosed?

A child psychiatrist or a specialist mental doctor diagnoses Conduct Disorders in children. Parents and teachers provide detailed insights into the child's behavior, which, along with observations and emotional testing, contribute to the medical diagnosis. If parents observe symptoms of Conduct Disorder in their child or teenager, seeking early treatment and assessment could be beneficial. Receiving treatment early can help avoid potential issues down the road.

Conduct Disorder frequently occurs alongside other mental health conditions such as mood disorders, anxiety disorders, posttraumatic stress disorder, substance abuse, attention-deficit/hyperactivity disorder, and learning disorders. This highlights the importance of early diagnosis and treatment. It's best to seek advice from your child's healthcare provider for further details.

## Conduct Disorder Treatment

The treatment for children with Conduct Disorders is determined by your child's doctor, taking into account factors such as age, health, wellness, and medical history.

### How severe are your child's symptoms?

Consider your child's tolerance for specific medications or therapies.

Anticipating the scope of the issue.

Share your thoughts or preferences.

***Treatment options vary from:***

Exploring cognitive-behavioural methods: The aim of cognitive-behavioral therapy is to enhance problem-solving abilities, communication skills, impulse control, and anger management skills.

Family therapy focuses on implementing changes within the family system, such as improving communication skills and family relationships.

Peer group therapy focuses on enhancing social and interpersonal skills.

When it comes to medication for conduct disorder, drugs may be considered if other symptoms or disorders could benefit from the medication, regardless of their effectiveness in treating conduct disorder.

Preventing Conduct Disorder in Children Similar to Oppositional Defiant Disorder (ODD), there is a school of thought suggesting that a series of challenges arise during the onset of Conduct Disorder. It may begin with inadequate parenting, along with academic struggles, and negative peer interactions. These interactions frequently lead to feelings of sadness and involvement with a rebellious social circle. Some other experts argue that various factors such as child abuse, genetic vulnerability, educational failure, brain damage, and distressing experiences play a role in the development of Conduct Disorder. Identifying and addressing negative family and interpersonal interactions early on can prevent the escalation of conflicts leading to disruptive and intense behaviors.

## Features of Conduct Disorders

A child with CD may exhibit a range of behaviors, from disobedience towards parents or authorities to truancy.

- Tendency to experiment with substances like cigarettes and alcohol at a young age.

- Showing a lack of empathy towards others.

- Behavior driven by spite and a desire for revenge.

- Showing hostility towards animals.

- Engaging in harmful behavior towards others, such as bullying and physical or sexual abuse.

- Tendency to become part of gangs.

- Enthusiastic about participating in physical altercations.

- Engaging in physical altercations involving weapons.

- Not telling the truth.

- Engaging in illegal activities like theft, arson, burglary, theft, domestic violence, and property damage.

- Struggling with learning.

- Struggling with low self-esteem.

- Struggling with suicidal thoughts.

Here is a link to other behavioral disorders: A child who develops Conduct Disorder typically exhibits irritability and temperamental behavior during childhood, although most challenging infants do not go on to develop Conduct Disorder. Oppositional Defiant Disorder (ODD) typically develops before Conduct Disorder (CD).

Consistent defiance, aggression, and outbursts are common traits of ODD.

Around 33% of children diagnosed with Conduct Disorder also have Attention Deficit Hyperactivity Disorder (ADHD). Depression affects 20% of children with Conduct Disorder. When a child is diagnosed with Conduct Disorder, it typically occurs between the ages of 10 and 16, with boys usually receiving the diagnosis earlier than girls.

## *Family influence:*

Disruptive behavior disorders have unclear origins, yet researchers suggest that family issues may contribute to the development of these disorders in children. Several factors contribute to a child's likelihood of developing Conduct Disorder:

### Parents struggling to manage their child's behavior.

Parents who fail to enforce consequences for their child's misbehavior, such as not following through on threats like restricting TV time, may struggle to see improvements in their child's behavior.

Insufficient supervision of the child's or adolescent's location by parents.

- Constant family disagreements.

- Living in poverty.

- Has a big family.

- Strict parenting, especially from the father.

- Marital discord.

- Domestic violence.

- Parents experiencing a mental condition.

- Parents who are concerned about illegal behavior.

- Child abuse.

- Surviving in institutionalized care and attention.

*Additional considerations:*

Additional elements that might play a role in the

emergence of Conduct Disorder or exacerbate its symptoms are:

- Boys are at a higher risk of having CD compared to girls.

- Peer group.

- Drug misuse.

- Dealing with mood disorders.

- Struggling with learning.

- Dealing with Post-Traumatic Stress Disorder (PTSD).

- Feeling down.

- Oppositional Defiant Disorder (ODD).

- Attention Deficit Hyperactivity Disorder (ADHD).

- Brain damage.

Here are some potential outcomes for children with Conduct Disorder if left untreated: - They may experience mental health issues, such as personality disorders, in adulthood.

- Feeling down.

- Struggling with alcohol addiction.

- Struggling with drug dependency.

- Living a lifestyle that involves breaking the law.

# What Leads to Conduct Disorders

Conduct Disorder highlights various issues without a specific known cause. It has been associated with:

- Child abuse and neglect.

- Parents abusing drugs or alcohol.

- Family discord.

- Strict or erratic discipline.

- Struggles with relationships and feeling excluded by peers.

- Experiencing assault or other traumatic events.

- Hereditary factors, such as a history of Antisocial Personality Disorder in parents.

- Living in poverty.

- Neuroimaging studies suggest that children with Conduct Disorder may develop brain abnormalities in certain areas. The pre-frontal cortex, responsible for our perspective, and the limbic system, influencing emotional responses, may be compromised.

- Research suggests that about half of anti-social behavior may be inherited through genetics. It remains unclear to experts what hereditary factors play a role in Conduct Disorder.

- Factors such as poverty, disorganized neighborhoods, family separation, parental psychopathology, harsh parenting, and lack of supervision are closely linked to Conduct Disorder.

- Children with cognitive deficits, such as low IQ, poor verbal skills, and impairment in professional functioning, may be more susceptible to developing Conduct Disorder.

**Who typically experiences conduct disorder?**

Boys are more commonly affected by the disorder than girls. Children diagnosed with Conduct Disorders often experience additional psychiatric issues that can play a role in the development of Conduct Disorder. Conduct Disorders are becoming more common in contemporary society among people of different races, ethnicities, and socioeconomic backgrounds.

# Chapter 2

## The signs of behavioral disorders

Conduct Disorder goes beyond typical teenage rebellion. This involves a significant behavioral condition that is likely to cause concern among educators, parents, peers, and other adults.

In order to receive a diagnosis of Conduct Disorder, children need to display a minimum of three symptoms within a year or at least one symptom within six months.

- Showing aggression towards individuals and animals.

- Bullies frequently use threats or intimidation towards others.

- Frequently instigates physical altercations.

- Frequently utilizes a tool that could lead to significant injury.

- Inflicting harm on individuals through physical means.

- Engaging in acts of physical cruelty towards animals.

- Taking without permission.

- Non-consensual sexual activity.

- Property Damage

- Intentionally starting a fire.

- Additional damage to property.

- Deception or Theft.

- Committing a burglary by entering a residence or stealing a car or items from a building.

- Deceiving others for one's own benefit.

- Taking items without facing the owner (like shoplifting).

- Committing a serious offense

- Staying up late or skipping school before turning 13

- Attempted to run away from home at night on multiple occasions • Frequently missing from school before the age of 13.

## Various Forms of Conduct Disorder

The DSM-5, utilized for diagnosing mental conditions, differentiates between Conduct Disorder with or without limited prosocial emotions. Individuals with insufficient prosocial emotions are often seen as lacking seriousness, being indifferent, and lacking empathy.

They may not prioritize their performance at school or work and exhibit superficial emotions. Their psychological expressions, when present, allow them to influence others.

## Conduct Disorder Impacts a Child's Functioning

Conduct Disorder impacts not only caregivers but also a child's functioning. Children diagnosed with Conduct Disorder often exhibit disruptive behavior that can impact their education. They may face disciplinary actions from teachers and have a tendency to skip school.

In addition, there is a high likelihood of them leaving school and struggling with interpersonal skills. Struggling to establish and nurture friendships is a common challenge for them. Family relationships often deteriorate because of their intense behavior.

Teenagers diagnosed with Conduct Disorder often face legal issues due to drug abuse, violent actions, and rule-breaking, which can result in incarceration.

They are at risk of acquiring sexually transmitted infections. Research indicates that adolescents diagnosed with Conduct Disorder may engage in sexual activity with multiple partners without using protection.

# Assessment of Behavior Problems

Diagnosing Conduct Disorder can be challenging due to its similarities with ODD and ADHD. Conduct Disorder can be accurately diagnosed by a child or adolescent psychologist, child psychiatrist, or pediatrician who specializes in behavior disorders.

Doctors could assess by observing and interviewing parents, the adolescent, and teachers. The teenager's actions are measured against a checklist in the Diagnostic and Statistical Manual of Mental Disorders published by the American Psychiatric Association. Conduct Disorder can be diagnosed if all necessary conditions are met.

## Therapy

Dealing with a child diagnosed with Conduct Disorder can be challenging due to their inherent distrust of unfamiliar individuals. We should consider the child's reluctance to follow rules. Identifying the numerous factors that influence a child's behavior may require some time.

Treatment options vary depending on the individual and may include the following:

- Counseling behaviorally.

- Cognitive Behavioural Therapy (CBT).

- Dealing with anger issues.

- Dealing with stress.

- Enhancing social skills.

- A unique educational initiative.

- Training for parents.

- Family therapy.

- Multisystemic therapy.

- Collaborated on a strategy involving family, teachers, and other care-givers.

- Addressing current issues.

- For individuals with a preexisting depressive disorder or ADHD, medication may be recommended.

### Where can assistance be found?

- Consult your doctor for any recommendations to a specialized service.

- Seek a child or adolescent psychologist.

## Key Points to Keep in Mind

Conduct Disorder is a behavioral condition found in children, characterized by hostility and a tendency to break rules. Behaviors involve avoiding pets and other individuals, engaging in illegal activities like setting fires on purpose, stealing from stores, and damaging property.

Treatment plans consist of behavioral therapy, psychotherapy, parental training, and family therapy.

# Assistance Tailored for Behavioral Disorders

Detecting Conduct Disorder and other related disorders early is crucial to offer your child a chance for early progress and a brighter future.

Given the seriousness of this disorder, the responsibilities can be divided among various environments, such as home, school, and community. The assistance offered is tailored to the child's growth, age, and situation.

It is crucial to engage and support the family. Focusing on strengths and identifying particular challenges for the young individual, like learning obstacles, can enhance outcomes for adolescents with Conduct Disorders.

Assistance with behavioral issues may include guiding the individual to enhance their positive, amicable actions, and manage their harmful antisocial behaviors.

### Assistance from the Comfort of Your Home

Parents and caregivers may find it challenging when a child exhibits oppositional or conduct issues. It's possible to feel apprehensive about your child and struggle with discomfort or even embarrassment regarding your child's condition. Feeling helpless and unsure about how to manage the situation is common.

It's common for parents to overlook their child's kindness and focus on their misbehavior instead. Over time, the child comes to the realization that attention is only received when rules are broken. Parents play a crucial role in showing care and support to their children, especially teenagers who may not always know how to seek it.

Being disregarded might lead to irritation or annoyance. Now you grasp how over time, a 'vicious reaction' is obtained.

Consistent and fair discipline is important when dealing with children. It's important for parents and caregivers to come to a consensus on disciplinary approaches and consistently show appreciation and affection.

It's challenging to accomplish on your own without support from others, and many parents/carers require additional assistance.

Parenting organizations provide the support and opportunity to connect with others facing similar challenges with their children. These groups are designed to help you encourage positive behaviors in your child.

### *Assistance for School*

Several adolescents facing behavioral challenges find it

difficult to cope in a school environment, causing them distress. Managing the school environment could assist in enhancing positive behaviors and boosting focus at home.

Adolescents struggling with behavioral issues often require support in developing social skills, which can be provided by schools. Certain children require specialized classroom assistance and assessment for learning challenges. If the issues are serious, certain children might need to be enrolled in specialized educational facilities to address their behavioral challenges.

### *Assistance from the community*

If the behavioral issues are significant and ongoing, or if there are concerns about Conduct Disorder, it's best to seek advice from your GP.

Specialist services are available to address antisocial behaviors. If specialized assistance is needed, they will suggest the local child and adolescent mental health service (CAMHS). This expert team collaborates with your child's school and other community organizations to support you and your child.

Experts are able to pinpoint the underlying issue and provide effective strategies to address the challenging behavior.

They can also provide assessments and treatments for other conditions that may arise concurrently, such as depression, anxiety, stress, and hyperactivity.

From social skills to behavioral therapy and talking therapy, the treatment covers a wide range. These therapies can assist a child in maintaining a positive attitude in various situations and improving their anger management skills.

# Chapter 3

## What Does Tantrum Mean?

When someone throws a tantrum, it's a brief display of anger through actions like crying, screaming, yelling, and tossing things around.

## What Causes Tantrums?

This is a common aspect of maturing. From ages one to four, many children may throw tantrums, but as they grow, they learn to become more independent. Children can get frustrated when they can't do something they want to do or are prevented from doing it. Struggling with independence versus frustration may result in tantrums.

Children may throw tantrums when they are tired, hungry, feeling ignored, worried, or stressed.

When a toddler is stressed, he may have difficulty communicating his feelings and may exhibit behaviors like crying, becoming clingy, and throwing tantrums.

# How to Handle Your Child's Tantrums

It can be quite distressing to hear your child's screams and yelling. Feeling upset, discouraged, and hopeless. Experiencing a tantrum in public or in front of others can be quite embarrassing. It's important to establish guidelines so your child can learn to navigate their emotions. It's typical for children to test limits frequently. These tips should help you effectively handle the situation with your child.

Stay calm instead of becoming upset. It's crucial not to panic. Just remember that it's completely normal, many parents go through this, and have confidence that you can handle it as well.

Ignore the outburst and carry on with your task calmly, whether it's conversing with someone, packing your groceries, or anything else. Remember to periodically check to make sure your child is safe. It can be challenging to ignore your child, but responding or even resorting to physical discipline can inadvertently reinforce their behavior.

Establish clear boundaries: You are determined to instill in your child the importance of rules and your commitment to upholding them.

When you notice signs of improvement, such as them no longer screaming, offer praise for their good behavior. Make sure to give your child your undivided attention, engage in warm and admiring conversations with them. By coming up with this innovative approach, you can help your child stay calm and well-behaved.

## How can I prevent tantrums?

Being prepared can help avoid tantrums by recognizing potential triggers or early signs of tantrum behavior in your child.

*Check out these examples:*

- Keep boredom at bay in a waiting room by bringing along your favorite books and toys to the hospital.

- Store favorite snacks out of sight, not within easy reach.

- Assist your child in regulating their energy levels by making sure they have scheduled naps rather than being awake all day.

- Address food cravings by providing a snack after school at 3.30 pm, rather than waiting until 5.00 pm for dinner.

- Consider using distraction as a strategy to prevent tantrums by redirecting your child's focus.

## Where can assistance be found?

It could be crucial to discuss it with parents, family, or friends. Consider discussing the issue with your child's teachers, as they may have encountered similar challenges at school.

If you're feeling worn down by tantrums, consider seeking advice from your family doctor, school nurse, or another healthcare professional. Parenting programs such as Triple P or Webster Stratton groupings are often found to be helpful by many parents and carers. At times, additional specialized support may be necessary for child and adolescent mental health services (CAMHS), particularly in situations involving significant stressors for a child, frequent tantrums, or self-harm behaviors.

# Assisting Your Kids with Behavioral Disorders

Common signs of Conduct Disorder in both children and adults include frequent walking away, cruelty towards people or pets, defiance, and irrational behavior. Although these behaviors may cause concern for parents, they can also lead to serious consequences for teenagers, such as suspension or expulsion from school or involvement in juvenile detention services.

Thankfully, medications in the early stages can have a beneficial impact on adolescents with Conduct Disorder. It's important to understand what signs to watch out for and the necessary actions to support your child effectively.

This concise guide aims to assist you in recognizing the indicators and understanding the necessary actions if you suspect your child has Conduct Disorder.

## Adolescent Conduct Disorder: Statistics and Facts

Among the general population, Conduct Disorder is more prevalent in boys than girls, with approximately 6 to 16% of children being affected.

- Children are more likely to develop Conduct Disorder if they grow up in urban areas rather than rural settings.

- Approximately 1% to 4% of children aged 9 to 17 are affected by Conduct Disorder.

- Conduct Disorder is a commonly diagnosed psychiatric disorder in children and adolescents in mental health settings.

- Conduct Disorder typically starts in childhood or

adolescence. "Child-onset" occurs before age 10 and is associated with a poorer prognosis compared to "adolescent-onset."

- Teenagers diagnosed with Conduct Disorder during adolescence are less likely to be later diagnosed with antisocial personality disorder after turning 18 compared to those with childhood-onset Conduct Disorder.

- Starting treatment for Conduct Disorder early increases the likelihood of success.

- Conduct Disorder is also known as disruptive behavior disorder.

## Dealing with Co-Occurring Disorders

- Additional mental health conditions that may be present before or alongside Conduct Disorder are:

- Attention-Deficit Hyperactivity Disorder (ADHD).

- Dealing with Post-Traumatic Stress Disorder (PTSD).

- Oppositional Defiant Disorder (ODD).

- Feeling down.

- Feeling anxious.

- Substance use disorders.

- Factors that increase the risk of Conduct Disorder: - A background of abuse or neglect.

- Experienced trauma in the past.

- Inherited tendency.

- Struggling academically.

- Experiencing a traumatic brain injury.

Searching for and Recognizing the Indications of Conduct Disorder

Identifying the signs early is crucial for getting your child the necessary support when dealing with Conduct Disorder. Signs of Conduct Disorder may involve hostility towards individuals.

- Instilling fear in others.

- Engaging in frequent conflicts with others.

- Showing cruelty towards animals.

- Causing harm to property, like starting fires.

- Telling untruths often.

- Taking without permission.

- Violating laws.

- Sexual assault.

- Often infringing on the rights of others.

- Frequently causing problems by making issues worse.

- Showing no regret for negative actions or causing harm to others.

- Struggling to understand or convey empathy.

- Breaking into people's homes or cars.

- Deceiving individuals.

- Consistently tries to intimidate others.

- Displaying aggressive behavior.

- Often disregarding the rules.

- Experiencing frequent challenges at school.

- Regularly absent from school.

- Physical altercations.

- Interpreting others as hostile or aggressive (when they're not).

- Struggling to understand public cues.

- Multiple injuries sustained from engaging in fights or experiencing accidents.

**Understanding the Initial Actions to Begin.**

If you suspect your teenager has Conduct Disorder, the initial three steps to address the issue are:

Step 1: Connect with your teenager by scheduling a one-on-one conversation to address your worries about their behavior.

Chances are, you've discussed this topic in the past, maybe during a moment of frustration or annoyance. Make sure your child knows you are there to support and motivate them to improve their behavior.

Given the significance of defiance in Conduct Disorder, it's likely that your child is reluctant to express it to you. Give him space, his true behaviors will show if they are there. Establish clear expectations and boundaries without resorting to yelling, lecturing, or power struggles.

Arrange a meeting for an evaluation: You can seek advice from your child's pediatrician or your family doctor. It's important to keep in mind that the individual does not have the expertise of a mental health professional specialized in treating complex disorders such as Conduct Disorder. A medical professional can conduct a physical examination to determine if there is a medical issue or substance abuse concern contributing to your child's challenging behavior.

It's crucial to have your child evaluated by a psychologist or psychiatrist, preferably a professional who focuses on working with children and teenagers. With their extensive background and expertise, these professionals can identify and comprehend the most intricate aspects of Conduct Disorder and its related issues. Consult your family doctor for suggestions.

Ensure your child receives treatment by taking the necessary steps. Therapy is the primary treatment for Conduct Disorder in teenagers, with the option of using medications to address co-occurring issues.

When it comes to treating Conduct Disorder, three highly effective types of chat therapy are cognitive-behavioral therapy (CBT), multisystemic therapy, behavior therapy, and family therapy.

Help your child recognize and transform negative thought patterns, self-talk, and beliefs with cognitive-behavioral therapy, a form of talk therapy that promotes healthy and positive thinking.

Multisystemic therapy is a comprehensive approach that requires active involvement from both the family and the community. It's advantageous for young offenders to deal with environmental elements such as family, educators, friends, and community.

Behavioral therapy aims to modify undesired behaviors by using positive reinforcement.

Family therapy, also known as functional family therapy, focuses on recognizing and altering detrimental family dynamics that could be exacerbating your teen's Conduct Disorder. Family therapy aims to decrease negativity in the household, boost support, and improve communication between family members.

Medication is not typically prescribed for treating Conduct Disorder, but it may be suggested to help alleviate symptoms of other conditions like ADHD, anxiety, or depression. It's crucial to handle children's medication with great caution due to their ongoing brain development. If your child's symptoms are moderate, the benefits far outweigh the potential risks.

Once your child is examined, suitable treatment plans will be recommended.

## Supporting and motivating your child

Supporting and encouraging an adolescent with Conduct Disorder can be challenging, especially when they display defiance or hostility.

Here are a few suggestions that might be useful:

- Make sure to educate yourself about Conduct Disorder to gain a deeper insight into your child's behavior and what they are experiencing.

- Consult with your child's therapist or psychiatrist for guidance on how to address aggressive, destructive, defiant, or cruel behaviors.

- Establish clear boundaries and guidelines in your household, while steering clear of power struggles with your child.

- Ensure you are available and willing to listen to your child, showing that you are always there to support them.

- It's important to be both fair and assertive when

setting and implementing rules.

- 6. Clearly outline the rules and the repercussions for not following them.

- Patience is key as your child works to change old habits and develop a better mindset.

- 8. Remember not to take your child's negative behavior personally.

- It's important to motivate your child to apply the skills they're learning in therapy while at home.

- It's important to recognize that Conduct Disorder is not something your child can simply overcome with willpower, nor is it just a phase of adolescence.

- Stay engaged in your child's treatment and communicate openly with the doctor about any questions or worries you may have.

- Strive to establish and uphold a calm and secure environment at home to assist in your child's treatment and overall mental well-being.

- Address undesirable behaviors in a structured and steady way without any unnecessary emotions.

- Strive to stay composed even in moments of fear or anxiety.

- 15. Show authentic support through both your words and actions.

- Make sure to regularly monitor your child's progress, assess the effectiveness of the treatment, and be ready to offer assistance whenever needed.

## Deciding the Best Course of Action when Situations Intensify

Raising children with Conduct Disorder can be challenging due to their impulsive and unpredictable behavior. This could lead to a rapid escalation and potentially result in a crisis. If your child has a tendency to harm family members, pets, classmates, or others, ensuring everyone's safety should be your top priority. Ignoring issues or expecting them to resolve themselves can result in serious consequences.

In case the situation worsens, it's important to seek help promptly. Reach out to your child's doctor promptly.

- Reach out to your close relatives or friends for assistance.

- Ensure to bring your child to the nearest medical center as soon as it is safe to do so.

## When Individual Therapy Falls Short

At times, individual therapy may not be sufficient to effectively address and control your teenager's Conduct Disorder. If your child exhibits behavior that is intimidating and poses a risk of harm to others.

- Threatening or planning suicide.

- Engaging in suicide gestures or attempts.

- Having difficulty managing tasks at home, school, or elsewhere.

- It may be time to explore an intensive treatment option. This may include intensive outpatient treatment (IOP) or psychiatric day treatment.

- Residential treatment available.

- Specialized treatment for individuals with co-occurring disorders.

- Treatment for psychiatric inpatients.

Intensive outpatient treatment or psychiatric day treatment can vary in the duration and frequency of sessions, such as twice a week or five days a week. Following these programs, regular outpatient treatment would consist of 1 hour of therapy several times weekly.

House treatment entails your child residing at a specialized non-hospital facility for adolescents with mental health disorders. Home treatment typically lasts for 30 to 180 days, depending on the condition and how severe it is. When dealing with drug abuse, opt for a residential program that offers comprehensive treatment.

Adolescents with Conduct Disorder and drug use

disorder should undergo dual diagnosis treatment. This treatment is typically conducted in a home treatment facility or an outpatient center.

For children who pose a risk to themselves and others, inpatient psychiatric treatment is often the most effective and intensive option available. Your child will need to be admitted to an adolescent psychiatric hospital for round-the-clock monitoring by medical professionals. This treatment typically extends over multiple days.

Every one of these immersive treatments offers daily therapy through various forms, including Individual and Group Therapy, as well as additional therapies like music therapy or art therapy. Your child may require regular or daily appointments with the doctor if they are still undergoing drug treatment.

## Self-Care Tips

Handling a teenager with Conduct Disorder can trigger a range of negative feelings. Various emotions can arise, such as hopelessness, helplessness, anger, disappointment, and despair. Feeling like a failure as a parent is common, often leading to self-blame for your child's behavior and reflecting on past mistakes. Being hard on yourself won't be productive, and it won't be good for your child either.

Given the impact of Conduct Disorder on your emotions, it's crucial to prioritize self-care. Proper self-care can ward off those negative emotions from overwhelming you and potentially enhance your mental health.

Here are some essential self-care steps to consider:

- Surround yourself with a positive and encouraging circle. This might involve your therapist, a pastor, and other individuals from your local church, local or online groups, family, and friends. Receiving ample support makes it simpler to motivate your child.

- Make sure to get enough rest and consume nutritious meals.

- Remember to prioritize self-care.

- Discover effective ways to manage your stress

levels.

# Chapter 4

## What is the definition of Conduct Disorder?

Children diagnosed with Conduct Disorder engage in physical fights, theft, and lying without feeling remorse or guilt if caught. They refuse to adhere to the rules and will not think twice about breaking them. They might start staying out late and skipping school.

Adolescents diagnosed with Conduct Disorder may also jeopardize their health and safety by experimenting with illegal substances or engaging in risky sexual behavior.

### How does this impact other people?

Conduct Disorder can cause significant stress for children, family members, universities, and the community. Children displaying such behavior may find it challenging to interact socially and struggle to grasp interpersonal dynamics.

Despite their potential, they struggle academically and

often rank low in their class. Deep inside, they may be grappling with feelings of inadequacy and self-doubt. It's common for them to become frustrated and point fingers at others when they struggle to work on self-improvement.

**What are the potential causes of Oppositional Defiant Disorder and Conduct Disorder?**

The cause of Conduct Disorder remains unidentified. We are starting to realize that there are various factors that can contribute to Conduct Disorder. If a child possesses certain genes that lead to antisocial behavior, they may be at risk of developing Oppositional Defiant Disorder/Conduct Disorder.

- Struggling to grasp appropriate social norms and behaviors.

- Display a strong temperament.

- Individuals with learning or reading difficulties may struggle to grasp lesson content, leading to frustration, self-consciousness, and disruptive behavior.

- Feeling down.

- Have experienced bullying or abuse in the past.

- Struggling with being hyperactive can lead to difficulties with self-control, focus, and following rules.

- Living with unconventional adolescents who engage in substance abuse.

*Another consideration:* Males tend to exhibit more behavioral issues and Conduct Disorder compared to females. Factors related to parenting, such as discipline and family separation. Parents often overlook good behavior and are quick to criticize and condemn their children, making things more complicated.

## Long-term effects of conduct disorder

Individuals displaying symptoms of Conduct Disorder during childhood are more likely to be male and have Attention Deficit Hyperactivity Disorder (ADHD), along with potential cognitive challenges such as learning disabilities or reading difficulties. Behaviors that appear early on are more likely to be associated with criminal and aggressive behaviors. Furthermore, there is a possibility that the young individual may be prone to associating with negative influences and engaging in substance abuse.

## How can I assist you today?

It's crucial to detect Conduct Disorder and other related disorders early on to pave the way for improvement and a brighter future.

When it comes to the seriousness of the issue, treatment can be provided in various settings such as at home or in educational and communal environments. The assistance offered varies based on the child's growth, age, and situation.

By highlighting the benefits and pinpointing particular challenges faced by young individuals, like learning obstacles, it can enhance the outcomes for teenagers dealing with Conduct Disorders.

Assistance for behavioral issues involves encouraging the individual to enhance positive and amicable behaviors while managing their harmful antisocial behaviors.

## *Assistance from the comfort of your own home*

Parents and caregivers may find it challenging when a child is dealing with Oppositional Defiant Disorder or Conduct problems. It's possible to feel apprehensive about your child and experience discomfort or even embarrassment regarding your child's condition. It's common to feel overwhelmed and unsure of how to manage the situation.

It's common for parents to overlook their child's kindness and focus on their misbehavior instead. Over time, the child comes to the realization that attention is only received when rules are broken. Many children, even teenagers, rely on their parents to show them love and might not know how to ask for it.

Being disregarded might lead to irritation or annoyance. Now you see how over time, a 'vicious reaction' is obtained.

Consistent and fair discipline is important when dealing with children. It's important for parents and caregivers to come to a mutual agreement on disciplinary strategies and consistently provide praise and affection.

It's challenging to accomplish on your own without support from others, and many parents and caregivers require additional assistance.

Parenting groups can help you get the help you require and connect with other parents whose children are going through similar experiences. These groups can train you to motivate positive behaviors in your child.

### *School-based help*

Anxiety arises from the fact that many teenagers with behavioral issues have difficulties in school. Enhancing positive behaviors and boosting focus at home could be achieved through school management.

Adolescents struggling with behavioral issues often require support in developing social skills, which can be provided by schools. Certain children require specialized classroom assistance and assessment of academic challenges. If the issues become serious, certain children may need to be placed in specialized educational facilities to address their behavioral challenges.

### *Assistance rooted in the community*

If the behavioral issues are significant and ongoing, or if there are concerns about Conduct Disorder, it's best to consult your GP for guidance.

Specialist services can help address antisocial behaviors. If specialized assistance is needed, they will suggest the local child and adolescent mental health service (CAMHS). This specialized team collaborates with your child's school and other community organizations to support you and your child.

Experts are skilled at pinpointing the underlying issue and offering effective strategies to address challenging behavior. They can also provide evaluations and treatments for other conditions that may arise concurrently, such as depression, anxiety, stress, and hyperactivity.

Various treatment options include social skills training, behavioral therapy, and counseling. These treatments could assist a child in maintaining composure in various scenarios and improving anger management.

# Chapter 5

## Conditions of Disruptive Behavior

Children diagnosed with Conduct Disorder often engage in physical fights, theft, and dishonesty without feeling remorse or guilt if they are caught. They refuse to adhere to the rules and will not think twice about breaking them. They might start staying out late and skipping school.

Adolescents diagnosed with Conduct Disorder may also jeopardize their well-being by experimenting with illegal substances or engaging in risky sexual behavior.

### How does this impact other people?

Conduct Disorder can lead to significant stress for children, family members, universities, and the community. Children exhibiting this behavior may find socializing challenging and struggle to grasp interpersonal situations.

Despite their potential, their academic performance tends to be below average. Deep inside, they may be grappling with feelings of inadequacy and self-doubt. It's common for individuals to become frustrated and point fingers at others when they struggle to see ways to grow personally.

## What are the causes of Oppositional Defiant Disorder and Conduct Disorder?

The cause of Conduct Disorder remains unidentified. We are starting to realize that there are various factors that can contribute to Conduct Disorder.

If a child possesses certain genes linked to antisocial behavior, they might be at risk of developing Oppositional Defiant Disorder/Conduct Disorder.

- Struggle with acquiring proper social skills.

- Display a strong temperament.

- Individuals who struggle with learning or reading may find it challenging to grasp lesson content, leading to frustration, self-consciousness, and disruptive behavior.

- Feeling down.

- Have experienced bullying or abuse in the past.

- They tend to be hyperactive, leading to difficulties with self-control, focus, and following rules.

Living with unconventional adolescents who misuse drugs.

Additional considerations:

Boys exhibit a higher prevalence of behavioral problems and Conduct Disorder compared to girls. Factors related to parenting, such as discipline and family separation. Parents often overlook good behavior and are quick to criticize and condemn their children, making things more complicated.

## Long-term effects of conduct disorder

An individual displaying symptoms of Conduct Disorder during childhood is more likely to be male and have Attention Deficit Hyperactivity Disorder (ADHD), along with low intelligence such as a learning disability or specific reading difficulties. Behaviors that appear early on are more likely to be associated with criminal and assaultive behaviors. Furthermore, there is a possibility that the young individual may be prone to associating with negative influences and engaging in substance abuse.

## How can I assist you today?

It's crucial to detect Conduct Disorder and other related disorders early on to pave the way for improvement and a brighter future.

Regarding the seriousness of the issue, treatment can be provided in various settings such as at home or in educational and communal environments. The assistance offered varies based on the child's growth, age, and situation.

Highlighting the benefits and pinpointing particular challenges of the young individual, like learning obstacles, can enhance the outcomes for teenagers with Conduct Disorders.

Assistance for behavioral issues involves encouraging positive and friendly behaviors while managing destructive antisocial behaviors.

## *Assistance from the comfort of your home*

Parents and caregivers may find it challenging when a child has Oppositional Defiant Disorder or Conduct problems. It's possible to feel apprehensive about your child and experience discomfort or even embarrassment regarding your child's condition. Feeling helpless and unsure about how to manage the situation is common.

It's common for parents to overlook their child's kindness and focus on their misbehavior. Over time, the child comes to the realization that attention is only received when rules are broken. Parents play a crucial role in showing care and support to their children, especially teenagers who may be seeking guidance.

Being disregarded might lead to irritation or annoyance. Now you grasp how over time, a 'vicious reaction' is obtained.

Consistent and fair discipline is important when dealing with children. It's important for parents and caregivers to come to a consensus on disciplinary approaches and consistently provide praise and affection.

It's challenging to accomplish on your own without support from others, and many parents and caregivers require additional assistance.

Parenting organizations provide the support and opportunity to connect with others facing similar situations with their children. These groups are designed to help you encourage positive behaviors in your child.

### *Assistance provided at school*

School can be a challenging environment for many teenagers dealing with behavioral issues, causing them distress. Enhancing positive behaviors and boosting focus at home could be supported by school management.

Adolescents struggling with behavioral issues often require support in developing their social skills, which can be provided by schools. Certain children require additional class support and assessment for learning challenges. If the issues become serious, certain children may need to be placed in specialized educational or academic facilities to address their behavioral challenges.

## *Assistance from the community*

If behavioral issues are significant and ongoing, or if there are concerns about Conduct Disorder, it's best to consult your GP for guidance.

Specialist services can help address antisocial behaviors. If you need specialized assistance, they will suggest the local child and adolescent mental health service (CAMHS). This expert team collaborates with your child's school and other community organizations to support you and your child.

Experts are available to pinpoint the underlying issue and recommend effective strategies to address the challenging behavior.

They can also provide assessments and treatments for other conditions that may arise concurrently, such as depression, anxiety, stress, and hyperactivity.

Various treatment options include social skills training, behavioral therapy, and counseling. These treatments could assist a child in maintaining a positive attitude in various scenarios and improving his ability to control his anger.

# Problems with Avoidant Personality

Someone who struggles with social interactions and experiences persistent feelings of inadequacy may be diagnosed with Avoidant Personality Disorder (AVPD).

Avoiding criticism, rejection, and shame is a common instinct for many people.

Individuals with Avoidant Personality Disorder often experience discomfort in social situations. They carefully examine their weaknesses and errors, which makes them reluctant to initiate discussions that might result in feeling embarrassed or rejected. As a result, individuals may experience feelings of isolation and lack of engagement in both professional and personal connections. Individuals with AVPD tend to avoid self-promotion, find reasons to skip events, and feel too shy to engage in social opportunities.

### What Causes Avoidant Personality Disorder?

The cause of avoidance personality disorder is still unknown to researchers, but some believe it may be a result of both genetic and environmental influences.

Signs of AVPD may manifest in early childhood. Research asserts that children who have care-givers that lack devotion and encouragement often experience rejection and can be vulnerable to risk. So are children who are abused, neglected, and get poor treatment. In response to these treatments, these children may avoid socializing with others. Researchers believe that another factor could be a physical illness. And about 2.5% of the populace would be qualified to get an Avoidant Personality Disorder diagnosis. It is a chronic disorder that affects both men and women. The condition can develop in youth, and symptoms have been recognized in children as young as two years old. However, like other personality disorders, Avoidant Personality Disorder is also diagnosed in adults.

**Avoidant Personality Disorder Symptoms**

Avoidant Personality Disorder has three major

components:

- Social inhibition.

- Feelings of inadequacy.

- Being sensitive to criticism and rejection

To get a diagnosis, an individual must have experienced these symptoms before early adulthood.

Besides, they need to manifest at least four of the following symptoms of AVPD:

- Avoiding activities at work that involves interpersonal contact because of the fear of being criticized or rejected.

- Unwillingness to connect with others unless they are sure they'll get a positive response

- Reluctant towards relationships because of the fear of being embarrassed.

- Worried about criticism in public gatherings.

- Feel uncomfortable in new social gatherings.

- Feel incompetent, unappealing, and inferior.

- Reluctant to take risks or engage in activities that can lead to embarrassment.

A diagnosis will require a psychological evaluation done by a mental doctor. This evaluation may eradicate potential diagnoses or determine whether you have other disorders.

## What is Cluster C Personality Disorder?

Different personality disorder diagnoses are organized in groups, or "clusters." Cluster C personality disorders are conditions where people involved are stressed or fearful. An avoidance personality disorder is a Cluster C personality disorder, as well as reliant personality disorder and obsessive-compulsive personality disorder.

## Is Avoidant Personality Disorder the same as Social Anxiety?

Researchers and doctors believe that Avoidant Personality Disorder only occurs with social anxiety disorder (SAD). However, latest research asserts that there is a large number of people with AVPD who do not meet the criteria to have public panic.

Sometimes it is challenging to discern whether you have social panic or Avoidant Personality Disorder, or both conditions. Usually, someone with AVPD will be anxious and avoid distressing situations. Whereas a person with interpersonal anxiety may have worries peculiar to certain situations, such as public presentation, and public speaking and performance.

To further differentiate between social panic and Avoidant Personality Disorder; people with Avoidant Personality Disorder may have co-occurring conditions such as depression, obsessive-compulsive disorder, or other personality and anxiety disorder. People with AVPD are vulnerable to drug abuse or suicidal behavior.

Sometimes Avoidant Personality Disorder can be confused with schizoid personality disorder, as both conditions involve public isolation. People with schizoid personality disorder are disinterested in interacting with others, while people with Avoidant Personality Disorder want relationships, they are often reluctant due to being scared of rejection or criticism.

## Treatment for Avoidant Personality Disorder

People who have Avoidant Personality Disorder may seek treatment because they wish to build stronger relationships with others and reduce the amount of stress they experience with everyone or at work. Coping with any personality disorder could be difficult, as one must have exhibited several symptoms for long.

Psychotherapy, or chat therapy, maybe the first Avoidant Personality Disorder treatment. Psychotherapy includes cognitive-behavioral therapy, which aims to reduce negative thought patterns and build social skills. Sometimes group therapy may be used to support individuals who have similar difficulties and create a haven for friendly interactions. Family therapy may also be useful so families understand the problem and provide a supportive environment that promotes development and good health.

There may be little or no research explaining the

effectiveness of drugs in treating Avoidant Personality Disorder. Sometimes drugs allow you to manage symptoms of Avoidant Personality Disorder or the symptoms of co-occurring disorders. Medications typically include antidepressants (i.e., selective serotonin reuptake inhibitors) and anti-anxiety medications.

**Getting Help for Avoidant Personality Disorder**

If you are reluctant to face crowds, or you feel awkward in public gatherings, this might spur you into thinking you have Avoidant Personality Disorder. It's important that you don't become afraid; you can get the needed help. The first step in getting help is by consulting a medical or mental doctor who can assess and diagnose you.

Therapy in a safe and warm environment can help you get over the anxiety you experience in public gatherings, including your fear of being rejected or criticized.

Also, your therapist can help you challenge negative values and explore the tiny but significant actions you can take to build solid relationships, be more involved at work, and establish romantic relationships.

# Understanding Personality Disorders and Suggestions for Managing Each Type

People struggling with stress and interpersonal challenges may be experiencing personality disorders.

Personality disorders are categorized in the Diagnostic and Statistical Manual of Mental Disorders (DSM) by the American Psychiatric Association as mental conditions. They are characterized by challenges in managing everyday stress and forming connections with family, friends, and coworkers, which may indicate a personality disorder. Individuals with personality disorders may not appreciate friendly gestures and might not realize they are exacerbating their issues.

Although each person has unique traits, personality disorders share certain common characteristics.

According to Scott Krakower D.O, an Associate unit central of psychiatry at Zucker Hillside Medical center in Glen Oaks, NY, all personality disorders consist of a behavior pattern that differs from cultural norms. Distortions in cognition, shifts in attitudes, and difficulties with social interactions and impulse control may be observed.

Aligned with Mental Health America, personality disorders fall into three distinct categories:

***Cluster A:*** Characterized by odd or eccentric behavior.

***Cluster B:*** involves dramatic, emotional, or erratic behavior.

***Cluster C:*** involves behaviors characterized by anxiety and fear.

Dealing with personality disorders involves helping the individual recognize and agree to treatment. According to Dr. Krakower, individuals with personality disorders could greatly improve with targeted therapies. Yet, they have the option to forgo treatment altogether or seek help only when the symptoms deteriorate.

Individuals with personality disorders often receive diagnoses such as substance abuse disorder, stress, and despair, according to Shawna Newman, MD, an adult, child, and adolescent psychiatrist at Lenox Hill Infirmary in NY. "If individuals have a personality disorder, they will face significant challenges," she remarks. While their condition can be controlled with treatment, completely getting rid of a personality disorder can be quite challenging or even impossible. Psychosocial interventions are frequently suggested for individuals with personality disorders, as Newman points out that there are no FDA-approved medications available for treating these conditions.

If multiple family members have a disorder, it's natural to feel concerned about your own risk, but it's important not to jump to conclusions.

"Certain health conditions may be hereditary, making other family members susceptible, such as diabetes or heart disease," explained John M. Oldham, MD, who holds key positions at the Menninger Medical Center and Baylor University of Medicine in Texas. There is a possibility of developing a personality disorder without showing symptoms during childhood if there was a disconnection in your bond while growing up.

According to Dr. Oldham, individuals with personality disorders may struggle to emulate others. "There's a stigma attached to every mental disorder, but there's also increasing awareness and research being done," he mentions.

Below is a summary of the ten personality disorders as outlined in the Diagnostic and Statistical Manual of Mental Disorders.

Borderline Personality Disorder is characterized as an instability in human relationships, self-image, and impulse control, according to the DSM. According to Dr. Krakower, they struggle with low self-esteem and face challenges in forming and sustaining relationships.

Nevertheless, they can find value in treatments such as dialectical behavior therapy (DBT). DBT involves a cognitive-behavioral treatment that integrates psychotherapy with group sessions to teach individuals new skills and techniques for handling emotions and addressing life challenges.

According to Dr. Oldham, while medication can aid in relaxation, psychotherapy is more effective. "With the right therapist and persistence, individuals with personality disorders have a great chance of making progress," he explains.

According to Dr. Oldham, individuals with borderline personality disorder often fear that they are not well-liked by others.

"The intensity of this feeling can lead them to argue with someone about their feelings or thoughts, even if the other person wasn't thinking about them at first," he explains.

"Their romantic relationships often face challenges due to their insecurities." Individuals with borderline personality disorder often display antagonistic and antisocial behaviors and may harm themselves through hitting or burning.

Individuals with Paranoid Personality Disorder struggle to trust others, typically beginning in early adulthood, according to Dr. Krakower.

"Moreover, they tend to be wary of others and often misinterpret innocent comments, always assuming that others are being dishonest," he elaborates.

According to the DSM, the disorder is characterized by a pervasive distrust and suspicion, where one consistently views others' intentions as malicious.

According to Dr. Newman, individuals with paranoid personality disorder often have unfounded suspicions. People often interpret innocent remarks in a negative way. They often misinterpret unintended insults and can be unforgiving.

Schizoid Personality Disorder: This disorder involves a disconnection from social connections and avoidance of others, according to the DSM. According to Dr. Krakower, most individuals tend to be more solitary and prefer activities done alone.

Individuals with schizoid personality disorder may find support through social interactions and organizations, yet they often avoid seeking treatment.

According to Dr. Krakower, Schizotypal Personality Disorder involves challenges in relationships, along with cognitive and perceptual distortions, and eccentric behaviors. "The typical person may hold superstitious beliefs or unconventional ideas," he elaborates. Even with this disorder, individuals can find support in social groups and organizations, yet many choose not to seek treatment.

Individuals with this condition tend to be superstitious and experience significant dysfunction, according to Dr. Newman. Their behavior is influenced by unusual values, like discussing clairvoyance or telepathy. Individuals with this personality disorder often experience unusual thoughts," she explains. According to her, people are usually cautious around them, except for immediate family members.

Antisocial Personality Disorder: This disorder involves a pattern of behavior characterized by disregard for and violation of the rights of others. According to Dr. Krakower, their disregard for public laws may result in multiple arrests and legal issues. "They might end up in jail," he elaborates. According to Dr. Oldham, individuals with antisocial behavior often exhibit a pattern of rule-breaking, disregard for codes of conduct, and manipulative and reckless tendencies. "They exhibit a lack of remorse for their actions and disregard interpersonal norms," he remarks. "Effective treatment for Antisocial Personality Disorder is currently unavailable, so prevention from childhood is crucial since correction becomes challenging once the disorder is established."

According to Dr. Krakower, individuals with Histrionic Personality Disorder often display attention-seeking behaviors, such as heightened drama and inappropriate intimacy or provocative actions. Occasionally, individuals may also be diagnosed with Borderline Personality Disorder. DBT therapy can provide significant benefits and support for individuals.

Exhibiting inflated behaviors with an exaggerated sense of one's personality is a characteristic of narcissistic personality disorder, according to Dr. Krakower. "Engrossed in unrealistic images of power and success, they frequently perceive others as inferior," he explains.

Individuals with this disorder exhibit a belief in their own uniqueness and seek excessive admiration from others. They often lack empathy and fail to consider the feelings of others," according to Dr. Oldham.

Individuals with a narcissistic personality disorder may also exhibit symptoms of borderline personality disorder and could benefit from therapy, according to experts. Unfortunately, many of them are reluctant to pursue treatment.

Behaviors associated with Avoidant Personality Disorder involve a strong tendency to avoid social interactions and a persistent feeling of being unwanted by others, according to Dr. Krakower. According to the DSM, the average person experiences feelings of inadequacy and is highly sensitive to criticisms. "It can be challenging for others to recognize if their family member or friend is dealing with this disorder," according to Dr. Oldham.

Psychotherapy is often the main form of treatment, according to him.

Person with Reliant Personality Disorder exhibits behaviors linked to excessive neediness or clinginess, along with fears of separation, according to Dr. Krakower.

Individuals with anankastic (obsessive-compulsive) personality disorder exhibit a strong inclination towards orderliness and perfectionism, often demonstrating inflexibility and rigidity, as emphasized by Dr. Krakower. Individuals with this condition struggle to part with possessions, even if they hold minimal emotional significance, according to experts.

# Chapter 6

## The disorder known as antisocial personality disorder

Antisocial Personality Disorder involves a persistent pattern of disregarding and violating the rights of others.

Understanding the disorder is enhanced when viewed within the realm of personality disorders.

This personality disorder involves persistent behavior that goes against universally accepted laws and norms. Typically, it begins in childhood or early adulthood, becomes a regular occurrence over time, and eventually results in personal issues or harm.

Symptoms of Antisocial Personality Disorder can vary in severity. Behavior patterns that are considered egregious or dangerous are often labeled as sociopathic or psychopathic. When someone has sociopathy, it means their conscience is impaired, while psychopathy is characterized by a lack of empathy towards others. Some experts characterize individuals exhibiting these symptoms as emotionally detached from the rights of others. The disorder can lead to various consequences such as imprisonment, drug abuse, and alcoholism.

Individuals with this disorder have the potential to achieve great things, but often struggle with feelings of irritability, hostility, and irresponsibility. They may experience multiple suicidal thoughts and could even make an attempt. It's challenging to tell when they're being deceitful or honest because of their manipulative nature.

Antisocial Personality Disorder is rarely diagnosed in individuals under 18, but symptoms of Conduct Disorder may appear before age 15.

Men are more likely to have Antisocial Personality Disorder than women. Men are more prone to Antisocial Personality Disorder than women. They often struggle with substance abuse and may be incarcerated or living in criminal environments.

### Signs of illness

As per the DSM-5, key characteristics of Antisocial Personality Disorder involve infringing on the physical or emotional rights of others.

- Dealing with instability in both personal and professional life.

- Feeling easily annoyed and displaying aggressive behavior.

- Showing no regret

- Consistent lack of responsibility.

- Being reckless and impulsive.

- Deception.

An evaluation has confirmed the presence of an antisocial personality. It is important to rule out other disorders before diagnosing APD.

Alcohol and drug abuse are prevalent among individuals with Antisocial Personality Disorder and can exacerbate symptoms of the disorder. Dealing with both substance abuse and Antisocial Personality Disorder simultaneously can make treatment more complex.

## *Reasons*

Given the uncertainty surrounding the disorder's origins, researchers have pointed to a combination of environmental and genetic influences. Suspected to be the root of antisocial behavior, hereditary plays a significant role. Individuals with biological parents displaying such behaviors are highly susceptible to inheriting and displaying them as well.

Environmental factors play a role as well; individuals may adopt antisocial traits if their role model exhibits them.

Around 3% of men and 1% of women are diagnosed with Antisocial Personality Disorder.

## *Therapy*

Dealing with Antisocial Personality Disorder can pose significant challenges. As symptoms of the disorder worsen in a person's life starting in their early 20s, individuals may notice a significant improvement in these symptoms by the time they reach their 40s.

Therapy, such as psychotherapy or chat therapy, is typically suggested for Antisocial Personality Disorder. Therapists are skilled at assisting individuals in handling negative behaviors and developing the social skills they may be missing. Typically, the initial step involves minimizing impulsive behaviors that could lead to legal trouble or harm. Utilizing family therapy can effectively educate the family members and enhance communication, while group therapy can be beneficial when surrounded by individuals facing similar challenges.

No medications have been approved by the U.S. Food and Drug Administration for treating Antisocial Personality Disorder. Medications might be suggested to help decrease intense or impulsive behaviors. They may also be prescribed to help stabilize moods or as antidepressants.

Any ongoing problems must be addressed as part of treatment, and they frequently include borderline personality disorder, attention-deficit/hyperactivity disorder, and disorders of impulse control as gaming disorder or sexual disorders. Individuals diagnosed with Antisocial Personality Disorder often struggle with substance abuse issues. The initial step in treatment involves stopping drug or alcohol use, followed by addressing substance abuse and personality disorder simultaneously.

Dealing with Antisocial Personality Disorder can be quite challenging. People rarely choose to pursue treatment on their own and typically only begin therapy when required by a court.

Antisocial Personality Disorder does not have a specific treatment.

Recently, there have been promising results with the antipsychotic medication clozapine in improving symptoms in men with Antisocial Personality Disorder.

## When can Antisocial Personality Disorder be diagnosed?

To receive a diagnosis of Antisocial Personality Disorder,

an individual must be at least 18 years old. It's important to have evidence of certification for a medical diagnosis of Conduct Disorder before the age of 15, since many symptoms of both disorders overlap. If the behaviors can be linked to symptoms of schizophrenia or bipolar disorder, a diagnosis of Antisocial Personality Disorder may not be made.

## Dealing with someone who has Antisocial Personality Disorder

Dealing with a loved one who has an antisocial personality disorder can be quite disheartening. Keep in mind that the absence of remorse or empathy is a characteristic of the disorder and can guide you in setting practical goals for your loved one's progress.

Through proper treatment, individuals with Antisocial Personality Disorder can enhance their relationships, take responsibility, and show respect for others' rights. Not everyone may see it the same way, so the family needs to decide how they want to respond to this situation.

It's fascinating that individuals with Antisocial

Personality Disorder who are married often show improvement in their relationship with their spouse compared to others.

It's important to prioritize your wellbeing and safety when someone you care about has antisocial personality disorder.

If you suspect Antisocial Personality Disorder in yourself or a loved one, it's important to seek help from a medical or mental health professional without delay. They will offer guidance and connect you with the appropriate resources to assist you in addressing this matter.

# Disorders characterized by oppositional and defiant behavior

*Could you please explain what Oppositional Defiant Disorder (ODD) is?*

ODD is a behavioral disorder typically identified in childhood, characterized by an uncooperative and defiant attitude towards parents, peers, educators, and others. According to research, children with ODD tend to cause more distress or trouble to those around them rather than experiencing it themselves.

## How Did Oppositional Defiant Disorder Come About?

Although the cause of ODD remains unknown, two theories have been proposed to explain its development.

According to a developmental approach, issues arise in children at a very young age. Children diagnosed with Oppositional Defiant Disorder may struggle to detach from individuals they are emotionally connected to. The negative traits associated with ODD are seen as a result of unresolved developmental issues from early childhood. According to learning theory, the negative traits of ODD may stem from the use of unfavorable parenting techniques by parents and authority figures. When parents provide negative support, it can actually fuel oppositional behaviors in a child by giving them the attention, time, concern, and conversation they seek.

## Who typically experiences Oppositional Defiant Disorder?

Behavioral disorders are often the main factors leading to referrals to mental health services for children. Oppositional Defiant Disorder impacts a range of school children, with a higher prevalence among young boys compared to girls.

## What signs and symptoms are present in oppositional defiant disorder?

Many symptoms commonly observed in children with Oppositional Defiant Disorder can also be seen in children who do not have this disorder, particularly between the ages of three and the teenage years. Several kids display these behaviors when they're tired, hungry, or irritated. They often display disobedience by arguing with parents or defying authorities.

Yet, in kids diagnosed with Oppositional Defiant Disorder, these signs appear often, impacting their learning and occasionally their interactions with others.

- Symptoms of Oppositional Defiant Disorder include frequent tantrums.

- Engaging in intense debates with adults.

- Not following adult instructions.

- Always challenging guidelines and refusing to obey rules.

- Always causing frustration or even provoking adults.

- Pointing fingers at others for their misbehaviors or mistakes.

- Gets easily irritated by others.

- Often displaying a hostile demeanor.

- Speaking in a harsh or unkind manner.

- Looking to get even.

ODD symptoms can mimic other medical conditions or behavioral issues. It's important to consult with your child's doctor for an evaluation.

## How Is a Doctor Diagnosed for Oppositional Defiant Disorder?

Adults such as parents, teachers, and other significant figures in a young person's life are usually the ones to recognize ODD in a child or adolescent.

Typically, ODD in children is diagnosed by a child psychiatrist or a specialist mental doctor. Parents and educators provide detailed insights into the child's behavior, along with medical observations and occasional mental testing, all of which play a role in the medical diagnosis.

If parents notice signs of ODD in their child or teenager, it's important to seek assessment and treatment promptly. Getting treatment early can help avoid potential issues down the road.

Additionally, Oppositional Defiant Disorder frequently occurs alongside other mental health conditions such as mood disorders, anxiety disorders, Conduct Disorder, and attention-deficit/hyperactivity disorder. This underscores the importance of early detection and intervention. It's best to seek advice from your child's healthcare provider for further details.

## Intervention for Oppositional Defiant Disorder

The treatment for children with Oppositional Defiant Disorder will be determined by your child's doctor.

- Consider your child's age, health, wellness, and medical history.

- How severe are your child's symptoms?

- Consider your child's tolerance for specific medications or therapies.

- Anticipating the extent of the issue.

- Share your thoughts or preferences.

Treatment options include individual psychotherapy, which focuses on cognitive-behavioral techniques to enhance problem-solving, communication, impulse control, and anger management.

Family therapy focuses on implementing changes within the family system, like improving communication skills and family relationships.

Raising children with ODD can be incredibly challenging and requires a lot of patience. Parents require assistance, empathy, and guidance in enhancing their parenting skills.

Peer group therapy focuses on enhancing interpersonal and social abilities.

When it comes to medication for conduct disorder, it may be considered if other symptoms or disorders could benefit from the treatment, regardless of its effectiveness against conduct disorder.

**Preventing Oppositional Defiant Disorder in Children**

According to some experts, a series of encounters are involved in the development of Oppositional Defiant Disorder. It often begins with inadequate parenting, combined with academic struggles, and difficulties in peer interactions. As these encounters progress, oppositional and defiant behaviors become a means of accomplishing tasks.

Identifying and addressing negative family and social interactions early can prevent the development of conflicts leading to oppositional and defiant behaviors.

Identifying issues early and providing treatment to enhance communication, parenting, conflict resolution, and anger management skills can help prevent negative behaviors and minimize the impact of oppositional and defiant behaviors in relationships with adults and peers, even in college and social settings.

Early treatment aims to enhance the child's healthy development and enhance the quality of life for children with Oppositional Defiant Disorder.

# Acknowledgements

Behold the magnificent triumph of this extraordinary book, a testament to the divine intervention of God Almighty and the unwavering love and support of my cherished Family, devoted Fans, avid Readers, loyal Customers, and dear Friends. Their ceaseless encouragement has paved the way for this resounding success.

www.ingramcontent.com/pod-product-compliance
Lightning Source LLC
Chambersburg PA
CBHW031131020426
42333CB00012B/323